Chair Yoga for Weight Loss

A Beginner Guide

copyrighted@2024

Justin Sky

Table of Contents

Chapter One

Chair Yoga
Introduction to Chair Yoga

Welcome to the world of Chair Yoga, where the benefits of yoga are combined with the comfort and accessibility of a chair. In this introduction, we will embark on a journey that redefines what it means to practice yoga, especially when it comes to weight loss goals.

Yoga has long been celebrated for its ability to improve physical, mental and emotional well-being. However, the idea of twisting into complex positions on a mat can seem daunting to many, especially those with limited mobility or physical challenges. That's where chair yoga comes in.

Chair yoga offers a gentle yet effective approach to yoga practice, making it accessible to individuals of all ages, fitness levels and physical abilities. By using a chair as a supportive prop, Chair Yoga allows practitioners to experience the benefits of yoga without having to lie down on the floor. This accessibility opens the door to a wider audience, including those who may have felt excluded from traditional yoga classes.

One of the most important advantages of chair yoga is its versatility. Whether you're looking to improve flexibility, build strength, reduce stress, or, as we'll explore in this book, achieve your weight loss goals, chair yoga offers a variety of techniques and poses that can be adapted to your specific needs and abilities. .

In this book, we delve into the principles of chair yoga, explore how it can support your weight loss journey, and provide practical advice on how to get started with your practice. From simple stretches to more dynamic sequences, discover how chair yoga can help transform your body and mind from the comfort of your own seat.

So, whether you're a seasoned yogi looking for a new approach or someone who's interested in yoga but hesitant to give it a try, I invite you to join me on this empowering chair yoga weight loss journey. Let's embark together on a journey of self-discovery, healing and transformation.

Principles of Chair Yoga

Exploring the Basic Principles of Yoga

Exploring the fundamental principles of yoga provides insight into its ancient wisdom and timeless teachings. These principles, often referred to as the "eight limbs" of yoga as outlined by the sage Patanjali in the Yoga Sutras, serve as a guide to living a meaningful and fulfilling life. Here's an overview:

1. Yamas (Ethical Guidelines): Yamas are moral and ethical principles that govern how we interact with the world around us. They contain:

   - Ahimsa (Non-Violence): Cultivating compassion and kindness towards self and others.

- Satya (Truthfulness): To speak and live truthfully, with integrity and authenticity.

- Asteya (non-stealing): Respecting the property, ideas and boundaries of others.

- Brahmacharya (Moderation): The practice of self-control and conscious consumption of resources.

- Aparigraha (non-possessiveness): Letting go of attachments and living in simplicity.

2. Niyamas (Personal Observances): Niyamas are personal disciplines that promote

self-awareness and self-care.
They contain:

- Saucha (Cleanliness):
Cultivating purity and cleanliness
in body, mind and environment.

- Santosha (Contentment):
Finding gratitude and acceptance
for what is, rather than seeking
external validation.

- Tapas (Discipline): Cultivating
inner strength, determination and
self-discipline to achieve your
goals.

- Svadhyaya (Self-Study):
Engaging in self-reflection,
introspection and study of sacred
texts to deepen self-awareness.

- Ishvara Pranidhana
(Surrender to a Higher Power):
Abandoning the ego and
surrendering to the divine will or
higher purpose.

3. Asanas (physical postures):
Asanas are physical postures
practiced in yoga. Although they
are often the most visible aspect
of yoga in Western culture, they
are only one component of a
holistic yoga practice. Asanas
promote strength, flexibility,
balance and relaxation in the
body, preparing it for meditation
and spiritual growth.

4. Pranayama (Breath Control):
Pranayama involves breath

control techniques that regulate the flow of prana (life force energy) in the body. Through conscious breathing practices such as deep breathing, alternate nostril breathing, and breath retention, practitioners enhance vitality, calm the mind, and connect with their inner essence.

5. Pratyahara (withdrawal of the senses): Pratyahara is the practice of withdrawing the senses from external distractions and turning inward. By redirecting attention away from external stimuli, practitioners cultivate inner focus, concentration, and introspection,

laying the foundation for deeper states of meditation.

6. Dharana (Concentration): Dharana involves developing sustained concentration on a single point of focus, such as a mantra, image or feeling. Through focused attention, practitioners quiet the fluctuations of the mind and cultivate mental clarity, stability, and presence.

7. Dhyana (Meditation): Dhyana is the practice of meditation in which the mind becomes fully absorbed in the object of focus. In this state of deep concentration, practitioners

experience a profound sense of inner peace, oneness, and connection with the divine.

8. Samadhi (Union with the Divine): Samadhi is the ultimate goal of yoga in which the practitioner experiences a state of complete absorption and union with divine consciousness. It is a state of transcendence beyond the ego where the individual merges with universal consciousness and experiences profound bliss and liberation.

These basic principles of yoga provide a comprehensive framework for holistic living that encompasses physical, mental, emotional and spiritual well-being. By incorporating these principles into daily life, practitioners can cultivate greater awareness, harmony, and fulfillment, ultimately leading to a more balanced and meaningful existence.

Adaptation of Traditional Yoga Poses for Chair Exercises

Adapting traditional yoga poses for chair practice is a creative and effective way to make yoga accessible to individuals who may have mobility limitations, injuries, or other physical challenges. Here are some common traditional yoga poses and how they can be modified for chair practice:

1. Seated Mountain Pose (Tadasana):

   - Sit tall in a chair with your feet flat on the floor and your knees hip-width apart.

   - Ground through your feet and lengthen your spine, reaching the top of your head toward the ceiling.

   - Relax your shoulders down and back and place your hands on your thighs or knees.

   - Breathe deeply while contracting your core muscles.

2. Seated Forward Fold
(Paschimottanasana):

   - Position yourself on a chair's
edge, keeping both of your feet
hip-width apart on the ground.

   - As you inhale, lengthen your
spine, then as you exhale, bend
forward from your hips and keep
your back straight.

   - Place hands on thighs, shins
or ankles, depending on
flexibility.

   - Relax your neck and
shoulders and breathe deeply into
the section along the back of your
legs.

3. Seated Twist (Ardha Matsyendrasana):

- Sit tall in a chair with your feet flat on the floor and your knees hip-width apart.

- As you inhale, lengthen your spine, then as you exhale, twist your torso to the right, place your left hand on the outside of your right thigh and your right hand on the back of the chair.

- Keep your shoulders relaxed and your spine long and look over your right shoulder.

- Hold the twist for a few breaths and then repeat on the other side.

4. Seated Cat-Cow Stretch:

   - Sit tall in a chair with your feet on the floor and your hands on your thighs.

   - Inhale to arch your back and lift your chest (Cow Pose), open your heart towards the ceiling.

   - With an exhalation, we round the back and pull the chin towards the chest (Cat Pose), while engaging the core.

- Continue moving with your breath, fluidly between cat and cow positions to warm up your spine.

5. Seated Warrior Pose (Virabhadrasana):

- Sit tall in a chair with your feet hip-width apart and on the floor.

- Extend your right leg straight in front of you and keep your leg bent.

- Bend your left knee and place your left foot firmly on the floor.

- Inhale to reach your arms overhead, lengthening your spine.

- As you exhale, bend your elbows and bring your hands into a prayer position at the heart center.

- After a few breaths of holding the pose, switch sides.

6. Seated Tree Pose (Vrksasana):

- Sit tall in a chair with your feet on the floor and your hands on your thighs.

- Lift your right leg off the floor and place the sole of your right foot on the inside of your left calf or thigh.

- Find your balance and lengthen your spine, bringing your hands into a prayer position at the heart center.

- After a few breaths of holding the pose, switch sides.

7. Seated Sun Salutation (Surya Namaskar):

- Start sitting on the edge of a chair with your feet hip-width apart and your hands resting on your thighs.

- As you inhale, swing your arms above your head to lengthen your spine.

- Exhaling, bend forward and bring your hands to your feet or the floor.

- As you inhale, lift yourself halfway up, lengthening the spine.

- With an exhalation, fold forward again, then with an inhale, stretch your arms above

your head and return to the
starting position.

Chapter Two

Breathing Techniques for Relaxation and Mindfulness

Breathing techniques are an integral part of relaxation and mindfulness practices in yoga. They help calm the mind, reduce stress and promote a sense of inner peace and presence. Here are some effective breathing techniques for relaxation and mindfulness:

1. Deep abdominal breathing (diaphragmatic breathing):

- Sit comfortably in a chair with your feet on the floor and your hands on your stomach.

- Close your eyes and take several deep breaths, allowing your belly to expand as you inhale and contract as you exhale.

- Pay more attention to your deep belly breathing than your shallow chest breathing.

- Feel the gentle rise and fall of your abdomen with each inhale, and let any tension or stress melt away with each exhale.

- Continue deep abdominal breathing for several minutes, allowing you to relax more deeply with each breath.

2. 4-7-8 breathing (relaxation breath):

- Sit comfortably with your back straight and your hands on your thighs.

- Close your eyes and take a few deep breaths to get into a relaxed state.

- Inhale quietly through your nose for 4 seconds and fill your lungs completely.

- Hold your breath for 7 seconds.

- Exhale slowly and audibly through your mouth for 8 seconds and completely empty your lungs.

- Repeat the cycle for several rounds, focusing on the rhythm of your breath and allowing your body to relax deeply with each exhalation.

3. Alternate nostril breathing (Nadi Shodhana):

   - Sit comfortably in a chair with a straight back and relaxed shoulders.

   - With the palm pointing upward, place your left hand on your left knee.

   - Bring your right hand to your face and place your index and middle fingers between your eyebrows, leaning lightly on the third eye point.

   - Using the right thumb, gently close the right nostril and inhale deeply through the left nostril for 4 seconds.

   - At the top of the inhalation, close the left nostril with the ring finger, release the right nostril and exhale slowly and completely for 8 seconds.

   - Inhale through the right nostril for 4 seconds, then close the right nostril with the right thumb, release the left nostril and exhale for 8 seconds.

- Continue this alternating
pattern for several rounds,
focusing on the smooth flow of
breath and the balance of energy
between the left and right sides
of the body.

4. Box breathing (square
breathing):

  - Sit comfortably with your
spine tall and your hands resting
on your thighs.

  - Breathe in deeply through
your nose for 4 seconds and fill
your lungs completely.

  - Hold your breath for 4
seconds.

- Exhale slowly and completely through your nose for 4 seconds and completely empty your lungs.

- Hold your breath for 4 seconds.

- Repeat the cycle for several laps, keeping a steady and relaxed pace.

- Focus on the square shape of your breath pattern so that each inhalation and exhalation is smooth and even.

5. Counted breathing:

- Sit comfortably and close your eyes.

- Inhale slowly and deeply through your nose within 4 seconds.

- For four seconds, hold your breath at the peak of the inhale.

- Exhale slowly and completely through your nose within 4 seconds.

- For four seconds, hold your breath at the base of your exhalation.

- Repeat this cycle for several rounds, gradually increasing the length of the number of breaths as comfortable.

- Focus on the rhythmic pattern
of your breath and the feeling of
relaxation with each exhalation.

These breathing techniques can
be practiced alone or in
combination with other relaxation
and mindfulness practices such as
meditation or gentle movement
to increase their effectiveness.
Experiment with different
techniques to find what works
best for you and incorporate them
into your daily routine to promote
relaxation, reduce stress, and
develop a greater sense of
mindfulness and well-being.

Benefits of Chair Yoga for Weight Loss

Chair yoga offers several benefits that can support weight loss efforts, making it an affordable and effective option for individuals looking to improve their health and well-being. Here are some ways chair yoga can help you lose weight:

1. Increased calorie burn: Chair yoga involves gentle movements and poses that engage different muscle groups and promote calorie burning. While the calorie expenditure may be lower compared to more intense forms of exercise, regular chair yoga

practice can still help create the calorie deficit necessary for weight loss.

2. Improved metabolism: Regular physical activity, even in the form of gentle exercises like chair yoga, can help increase metabolism. By stimulating muscles and increasing heart rate, Chair Yoga promotes metabolic activity, which can improve the body's ability to burn calories and fat, supporting weight loss goals.

3. Muscle tone and strength: Chair yoga involves poses and movements that target different muscle groups, helping to

improve muscle tone and strength. Building lean muscle mass not only improves physical appearance, but also increases your metabolic rate because muscle tissue requires more energy to maintain than fat tissue. As a result, Chair Yoga can contribute to long-term weight management.

4. Stress Reduction: Stress is often a contributing factor to weight gain and difficulty losing weight. Chair yoga includes relaxation techniques such as deep breathing, mindfulness and gentle stretching that can help reduce stress levels and promote

relaxation. By managing stress more effectively, individuals may be less likely to engage in emotional eating or other unhealthy behaviors that sabotage weight loss efforts.

5. Improved digestion: Certain positions and movements in the chair can stimulate digestion and improve gastrointestinal function. By promoting movement in the abdominal area and promoting relaxation of the digestive organs, chair yoga can aid digestion and relieve symptoms such as bloating and discomfort, which can indirectly promote weight loss.

6. Mindful Eating: Chair yoga emphasizes mindfulness and awareness, both on and off the mat. Through mindfulness practices incorporated into chair yoga classes, individuals can develop greater awareness of their eating habits, including feelings of hunger and fullness, as well as emotional triggers for overeating. This mindfulness can lead to more conscious and balanced eating habits that promote sustainable weight loss.

7. Accessibility and Inclusivity: One of the significant advantages of Chair Yoga is its accessibility to individuals of all ages, fitness

levels and physical abilities. Whether someone is recovering from an injury, managing chronic pain, or struggling with limited mobility, chair yoga offers a gentle and supportive way to engage in physical activity and promote overall well-being, making it a viable option for those who may not be able to participate in traditional forms of exercise.

Overall, chair yoga can be a valuable tool in a comprehensive weight loss program, offering physical, mental, and emotional benefits that support healthy lifestyle changes and long-term weight management. By incorporating chair yoga into their routine, individuals can improve their overall well-being while working towards their weight loss goals in a sustainable and holistic way.

Chapter Three

Getting Started With Chair Yoga

Choosing the Right Chair and Exercise Space

Choosing the right chair and chair yoga space is essential to ensure comfort, safety and an enjoyable experience. Here's how to choose the right chair and create the ideal space for your workout:

1. Choosing a chair:

   - Choose a sturdy chair without wheels: Choose a chair with a stable base and a solid structure that will provide you with sufficient support during exercise.

Avoid chairs with wheels, as they may not provide the stability needed for certain positions.

- Choose a chair with a flat seat: Look for a chair with a flat and straight seat rather than a chair with a shaped or angled seat. The flat seat allows for a more comfortable and balanced sitting position during yoga poses.

- Consider armrests: While not necessary, chairs with armrests can provide additional support and stability, especially for those with limited mobility or balance issues.

- Ensure the correct height: The chair should be at a height that allows your feet to rest comfortably on the floor with your knees at a 90 degree angle. If necessary, adjust the height of the chair by adding cushions or pads.

2. Preparation of the space:

- Clear the area: Choose an area free of clutter and obstructions so that you have enough room to move comfortably. Remove any furniture or objects that could impede your movement or pose a safety risk.

- Use a non-slip surface: Place the chair on a non-slip surface such as a yoga mat or carpet to prevent it from sliding during exercise. This will ensure increased stability and safety, especially during dynamic movements.

- Create a soothing atmosphere: Get in the mood for exercise by creating a soothing and pleasant atmosphere in your exercise space. Dim the lights play soft music or nature sounds, and use essential oils or candles to increase relaxation and mindfulness.

- Consider privacy: Choose a quiet and private space where you can practice without distractions or interruptions. This allows you to fully immerse yourself in your practice and focus on your breath and movements.

Warm-Up Exercises to Prepare the Body

Warming up before chair yoga is important to prepare the body for movement, increase blood flow to the muscles and reduce the risk of injury. Here are some gentle warm-up exercises you can incorporate into your routine:

1. Seated Shoulder Roll:

- Sit comfortably in a chair with your feet on the floor and your hands on your thighs.

- Inhale and raise your shoulders towards your ears.

- As you exhale, rotate your shoulders back and down and press your shoulder blades together.

- Repeat this movement several times, letting your breath guide the movement of your shoulders.

2. Stretching the neck:

- Sit tall in a chair with a straight spine and relaxed shoulders.

- Inhale to lengthen your spine, then as you exhale gently tilt your head to the right and bring your right ear closer to your right shoulder.

- Hold the breath for several breaths and feel a gentle stretch along the left side of the neck.

- With an inhale return to the center, then with an exhale repeat the stretch on the left side.

- Continue alternating sides, moving with your breath and

maintaining gentle, steady pressure.

3. Seated cat-cow stretch:

   - Sit on the edge of a chair with your feet on the floor and your hands on your thighs.

   - Inhale and arch your back and lift your chest forward (Cow Pose), open your heart towards the ceiling.

   - Engage your core as you exhale around your spine and pull your chin to your chest (Cat Pose).

   - Move between cat and cow with your breath, moving slowly

and carefully to warm the spine
and stretch the back muscles.

4. Seated side stretches:

   - Sit tall in a chair with your
feet on the floor and your hands
on your thighs.

   - Inhale to lengthen your spine,
and then exhale to reach your
right arm overhead and lean to
the left, stretching the right side
of your body.

   - Hold the breath for a few
breaths and you will feel a gentle
opening along the right side of
the torso.

   - Return to the center with an
inhale, and then repeat the

stretch on the opposite side with an exhale.

   - Continue to alternate sides, move with your breath and maintain awareness of your alignment.

5. Seated forward fold:

   - Sit on the edge of a chair with your feet hip-width apart and your hands resting on your thighs.

   - Inhale to lengthen your spine, and then exhale as you bend forward from your hips and keep your back straight.

- Place your hands on your shins or ankles, depending on your flexibility.

- Hold the breath for several breaths and feel a gentle release along the back of the legs and spine.

- Inhale to slowly roll back into a seated position and straighten your spine one vertebra at a time.

These warm-up exercises gently mobilize the spine, shoulders, neck and hips, preparing the body for the more dynamic movements and stretches of chair yoga. Remember to move mindfully,

listen to your body, and adjust
exercises as needed to suit your
comfort and ability level.

Chapter Four

Chair Yoga Sequence for Weight Loss

Energizing Sequence to Boost Metabolism

Here's an energizing chair yoga sequence designed to boost metabolism and energize the body. These dynamic movements will increase blood circulation, stimulate the digestive system and awaken your energy. Remember to move with your breath and adjust positions as needed to suit your comfort and ability level.

1. Seated Mountain Pose (Tadasana):

- Sit tall in a chair with your feet on the floor and your hands on your thighs.

- Close your eyes and take a few deep breaths, ground yourself and set an intention for your practice.

- Inhale as you reach your arms overhead, lengthen your spine and lift your chest.

- As you exhale bring your hands back to your heart center, feeling strong and centered.

2. Seated Sun Salutations (Surya Namaskar):

- As you inhale, swing your arms above your head and lengthen your spine.

- Exhaling, bend forward and bring your hands to your feet or the floor.

- As you inhale, lift yourself halfway up, lengthening your spine.

- With an exhalation, fold forward again, then with an inhale, stretch your arms above your head and return to the starting position.

- Repeat the sequence several times, moving with your breath and fluidly between each position.

3. Seated chair pose (Utkatasana):

- Sit at the front edge of the chair with your feet hip-width apart and your knees aligned above your ankles.

- Inhale as you reach your arms overhead, lengthening your spine.

- Exhaling, you bend your knees and lower your hips towards the chair as if you were sitting in an invisible chair.

- Hold the pose for several breaths, engaging the core and thighs and keeping the chest lifted.

4. Seated twist with side bend:

   - As you inhale, lengthen your spine, then as you exhale, turn your torso to the right, place your left hand on the outside of your right thigh and your right hand on the back of the chair.

   - Inhale to lengthen your spine even more, and then exhale as you lean to the right, feeling a stretch along the left side of your body.

   - Hold the pose for a few breaths, and then inhale to return to center and repeat on the other side.

5. Seated warrior II
(Virabhadrasana II):

- Sit towards the front edge of
the chair with your feet wide
apart and your knees aligned
above your ankles.

- Inhale and stretch your arms
out to the sides, parallel to the
floor.

- As you exhale, bend your
right knee and turn your torso to
the right, looking through the tips
of your right fingers.

- Hold the pose for several
breaths, feeling strong and
grounded through the legs and
energized through the fingertips.

- Return to the center with an inhale, and then repeat on the other side with an exhale.

6. Seated dancing warrior (Natarajasana):

- Sit at the front edge of the chair with your feet hip-width apart and your hands resting on your thighs.

- With an inhale, raise your right knee to your chest and lift your right leg off the floor.

- As you exhale, extend your right leg straight in front of you, bend your leg and stretch your arms above your head.

- Hold the pose for a few breaths, feeling strong and balanced, then inhale and return to the starting position.

- Repeat on the other side, bringing the left knee up to the chest and extending the left leg forward.

7. Seated breath of fire (Kapalabhati Pranayama):

- Sit tall in a chair with your feet on the floor and your hands on your thighs.

- Take a deep breath in through your nose, then exhale forcefully through your nose and pump your belly in and out.

- Continue this fast, rhythmic
breathing for 30-60 seconds,
focusing on the feeling of warmth
and energy building in your body.

8. Seated relaxation pose
(Savasana):

  - Sit comfortably in a chair with
your feet on the floor and your
hands on your thighs.

  - Close your eyes and take a
few deep breaths to completely
relax your body.

  - With each exhalation release
any tension or stress and allow
yourself a few moments of
stillness to enjoy the energizing
effects of your practice.

Core Strengthening Poses for Toning

Core strengthening poses are excellent for strengthening the abdominal muscles and improving overall stability. Here are a series of yoga chair poses aimed at strengthening the core:

1. Seated spinal twist (Ardha Matsyendrasana):

   - Sit tall in a chair with your feet on the floor and your hands on your thighs.

   - As you inhale, lengthen your spine, then as you exhale, turn your torso to the right, place your left hand on the outside of your right thigh and your right hand on the back of the chair.

   - Keep your shoulders relaxed and your spine long and look over your right shoulder.

   - Engage your core muscles to encourage twisting, feel the gentle activation along the sides of your waist and abdomen.

   - Hold the pose for a few breaths, then inhale to return to center and repeat on the other side.

2. Seated boat pose (Navasana):

   - Sit towards the front edge of the chair with your feet flat on the floor and your knees bent.

- Hold on to the sides of the chair for support or extend your arms forward at shoulder height for an added challenge.

- Inhale to lengthen your spine, and then exhale to lift your legs off the floor, balancing on your sit bones.

- Engage your core muscles to stabilize your torso and lift your legs higher to form a "V" shape with your body.

- Hold the pose for several breaths and feel the deep activation of the abdominal and hip flexors.

- To adjust, keep your knees bent and feet on the floor and focus on engaging your core muscles.

3. Seated knee to chest pose:

- Sit tall in a chair with your feet on the floor and your hands on your thighs.

- Inhale to lengthen your spine, and then as you exhale, press your right knee to your chest and gently bring it in with your hands.

- Engage your core muscles to lift your knee higher toward your chest, feeling a deep stretch in your lower back and hip flexors.

- Repeat on the opposite side after holding the pose for a few breaths.

- For an added challenge, extend your opposite leg straight out in front of you, lifting it off the floor and bringing your knee to your chest.

4. Seated side plank (Vasisthasana):

- Sit towards the front edge of the chair with your legs straight and knees bent.

- Place your right hand on the seat of the chair and stretch your left arm towards the ceiling.

- Engage your core muscles and lift your hips off the chair to get into a side plank position.

- Keep your body in a straight line from head to toe and hold the pose for several breaths, feeling the strong activation of your obliques and core.

- To modify, bend the bottom knee and place it on the floor for more support, or keep both knees bent with the top leg in front of the bottom leg.

5. Seated leg lifts:

- Sit towards the front edge of the chair with your feet on the floor and your hands on your thighs.

- Inhale to lengthen your spine, then exhale and lift your right leg straight out in front of you, engaging your core muscles.

- Hold the pose for a few breaths and then lower the leg with control down.

- Repeat on the other side and lift your left leg straight out in front of you.

- Focus on maintaining stability in the trunk and pelvis as you raise and lower your legs, feeling deep activation in the lower abdomen.

6. Seated forward bend with twist:

   - Sit tall in a chair with your feet on the floor and your hands on your thighs.

   - Inhale to lengthen your spine, and then exhale as you bend forward from your hips and keep your back straight.

- Place your hands on your shins or ankles, depending on your flexibility.

   - Inhale to lengthen your spine even more, and then exhale, twist your torso to the right and place your left hand on the outside of your right shin.

- Hold the twist for a few breaths, feeling deep activation in your obliques and core, then repeat on the other side.

Gentle Stretch to Improve Flexibility and Mobility

Here's a gentle chair yoga sequence focusing on stretches to improve flexibility and mobility. These poses target different areas of the body, including the spine, hips, shoulders and legs, helping to release tension, increase range of motion and promote relaxation. Remember to move mindfully, breathe deeply and listen to your body during the sequence.

1. Seated neck stretch:

- Sit tall in a chair with your feet on the floor and your hands on your thighs.

- Inhale to lengthen the spine, and then as you exhale, tilt your head to the right and bring your right ear closer to your right shoulder.

- Hold the breath for several breaths and feel a gentle release along the left side of the throat.

- With an inhale return to the center, then with an exhale repeat the stretch on the left side.

- Continue alternating sides, moving with your breath and maintaining gentle, steady pressure.

2. Seated shoulder stretch:

- Sit tall in a chair with your feet on the floor and your hands on your thighs.

- Inhale to reach your right arm straight to the ceiling, then exhale, bend your right elbow and extend your right hand to your left shoulder blade.

- With your left hand, gently press the right elbow and deepen the right shoulder area.

- Hold the breath for a few breaths and you will feel a gentle opening across the front of your right shoulder.

- Inhale to release the stretch, then exhale and repeat on the left side.

3. Seated Spinal Twist:

- Sit tall in a chair with your feet on the floor and your hands on your thighs.

- As you inhale, lengthen your spine, then as you exhale, turn your torso to the right, place your left hand on the outside of your right thigh and your right hand on the back of the chair.

- Keep your shoulders relaxed and your spine long and look over your right shoulder.

- Hold the twist for several breaths and feel a gentle release along the spine.

- Inhaling, return to the center, then exhaling, repeat the twist on the left side.

4. Seat forward fold:

- Sit towards the front edge of the chair with your feet on the floor and your hands on your thighs.

- Inhale to lengthen your spine, and then exhale as you bend forward from your hips and keep your back straight.

   - Place your hands on your shins, ankles or the floor, depending on your flexibility.

   - Hold the breath for several breaths and feel a gentle release along the back of the legs and spine.

   - Inhale to slowly roll back into a seated position and straighten your spine one vertebra at a time.

5. Seated hip opener:

   - Sit tall in a chair with your feet on the floor and your hands on your thighs.

- As you inhale, lengthen your spine, then as you exhale, cross your right ankle over your left knee and bend your right leg.

- Keeping your spine straight and chest lifted gently push into your right knee to deepen the stretch in your right hip.

- Hold the breath for a few breaths and feel a gentle opening in the right hip and outer thigh.

- Inhale to release the stretch, then exhale and repeat on the other side.

6. Seated figure four stretch:

- Sit tall in a chair with your
feet on the floor and your hands
on your thighs.

- As you inhale, lengthen your
spine, then as you exhale, cross
your right ankle over your left
knee and bend your right leg.

- Keeping your spine straight
and chest lifted gently push into
your right knee to deepen the
stretch in your right hip.

- Hold the breath for a few
breaths and feel a gentle opening
in the right hip and outer thigh.

- Inhale to release the stretch,
then exhale and repeat on the
other side.

7. Seated hamstring stretch:

- Sit towards the front edge of the chair with your feet on the floor and your hands on your thighs.

- Extend your right leg straight in front of you and bend your leg.

- Inhale to lengthen your spine, and then exhale as you bend forward from your hips and keep your back straight.

- Place your hands on your right shin or ankle, depending on your flexibility.

- Hold the stretch for several breaths and feel a gentle release along the back of the right leg.

- Inhale to slowly sit up, then
exhale and repeat on the other
side.

8. Seated side stretch:

- Sit tall in a chair with your
feet on the floor and your hands
on your thighs.

- Inhale to reach your right arm
above your head, lengthening
your spine.

- As you exhale, lean to the left
and feel a gentle stretch along
the right side of your body.

- Keep both hips firmly on the
chair and avoid collapsing into a
stretch.

- Hold the stretch for a few breaths, and then inhale to return to center and repeat on the other side.

9. Seated calf stretch:

- Sit towards the front edge of the chair with your feet on the floor and your hands on your thighs.

- Extend your right leg straight in front of you and bend your leg.

- Inhale to lengthen the spine, then exhale, gently point your fingers to the ceiling and feel a stretch along the back of your right calf.

- Hold the stretch for a few
breaths, then inhales to release
and repeat on the other side.

10. Seated relaxation pose
(Savasana):

- Sit comfortably in a chair with
your feet on the floor and your
hands on your thighs.

- Close your eyes and take a
few deep breaths to completely
relax your body.

- With each exhalation release
any tension or stress and take a
few moments of peace and enjoy
the feeling of openness and
freedom in your body.

Chapter Five

Mindful Eating and Chair Yoga

Combining mindful eating with chair yoga can be a powerful way to cultivate awareness, nourish your body, and promote overall well-being. Here's how you can incorporate mindfulness practices into your meals and chair yoga practice:

1. Mindful eating:

   - Start by setting a conscious intention before you eat. Take a moment to express gratitude for the food you are about to eat and the nutrition it provides.

- Create a calm and pleasant environment to eat without distractions. Turn off electronic devices, eat at the table and enjoy every bite without rushing.

- Use all your senses to fully experience food. Notice the colors, textures and smells of the food. Take small bites and chew slowly, savoring the flavors and sensations in your mouth.

- Pay attention to hunger and satiety signals. Eat when you're hungry and stop when you're satisfied, listening to your body's signals rather than external signals.

- Practice mindful meditation
while eating by focusing your
attention on the sensations of the
food. Feel the movements of your
jaw, the taste of food, and
feelings of satisfaction as you
nourish your body.

- Cultivate gratitude for the
nourishment you receive from
food and the connection it fosters
with others. Share a meal with
loved ones and appreciate the
opportunity to bond and bond
over food.

2. Practicing yoga on a chair:

- Begin your chair yoga practice
with a few moments of mindful

breathing. Sit comfortably in a chair, close your eyes and take a few deep breaths to center yourself and bring your awareness to the present moment.

- Go through gentle chair yoga poses with an alert mind and focus on the sensations in your body and the rhythm of your breath. Notice any areas of tension or resistance and allow your breath to soften and release them.

- Practice gratitude and self-compassion as you move through your chair yoga practice. Appreciate your body's capabilities and respect its limitations, approach each pose with kindness and acceptance.

- Use your breath as an anchor to cultivate mindfulness during your practice. Notice the sensations of each inhale and exhale, allowing your breath to guide your movements and ground you in the present moment.

- Take moments of quiet and reflection between poses to check in with you and observe any changes in your body, mind and emotions. Notice how chair yoga affects your mood, energy levels, and overall sense of well-being.

- End your chair yoga practice with a few moments of gratitude and self-reflection. Take a moment to acknowledge that you are showing up and nurturing your body and mind through mindful movement.